Aena
&
604 743 2670 cel.
604 824-7775

ADRENAL FATIGUE

A DESK
REFERENCE

SALMAAN DALVI
(PhD. Nutritional Medicine)

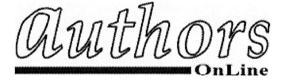

Visit us online at www.authorsonline.co.uk

An AuthorsOnLine Book

Published by Authors OnLine Ltd 2003

ISBN 0-7552-0093-4

Authors OnLine Ltd
Hertford
England

This book is also available in e-Book format from
www.authorsonline.co.uk

Acknowledgements

This work would never have been completed without the encouragement of many special people. My gratitude goes out first to all my clients, teachers, colleagues, family and friends.

I gratefully acknowledge the following people for their role in making my work a reality and at times by pushing me to carry on writing when I was down and suffering Adrenal Fatigue myself.

Firstly both my parents who have been a great moral and emotional support throughout my life. My success in life is as a result of their hard work and emphasis on education.

The late Mr. N.C, Haji and Mr. M.M. Patel who were my teachers in Tanzania and gave me the foundation required to study alternative medicine with a scientific approach.

Mr. Ali Alekar for teaching me chemistry.

My thanks and gratitude to my best friend Dr. M. Kauchali who has been a towering support whenever I needed help whether it was my computer crashing or reviewing medical facts.

I owe so much to so many people who I have not named in the book but who have been a constant source of encouragement and support. My special thanks and appreciation goes to a wonderful individual who will always be a part of my life no matter what physical and emotional distances separate us.

DEDICATED TO

My Great Uncle

Muhammad Saleh Mahmood Dalvi

of

Dhabil, District Ratnagiri, Maharashtra, India.

In Fond memory of his contribution to Ayurveda and
Homeopathy as a practitioner for over fifty years.

ABOUT THE AUTHOR

Salmaan Dalvi, (PhD. Nutritional Medicine) is a well-known nutritionalist, TV Health Presenter and lifestyle management consultant, with extensive experience in natural and complementary medicine. Dr. Dalvi is an international speaker, lifestyle coach and health and wellness consultant and appears regularly on radio and television programs.

Following a career in research and development of herbal nutritional products, he now develops and researches products that enhance quality of life. He specialises in Food intolerance, Hormonal imbalances and vitamin and mineral deficiency testing, using the Bio-Energetic Stress Testing. He works with a computer based electro-dermal therapeutic device, which enables him to test and detect subtle energy changes and dysfunctions in the human body and estimates the extent of pathological processes within diseased organs, by depicting energy imbalances at acupressure points. His knowledge of herbal and nutritional supplements assists him in providing individualised supplementation protocols to correct imbalances and deficiencies. Dr. Dalvi has been involved in the research and development of three breakthrough formulations, in South Africa and UK.

The author of the book intends to use a percentage of the revenue generated from the sale of the book towards development of Nutritional Health centres in Southern Africa.

FOREWARD

by

Dr. Martin Dodds

Every Science student learns that the function of the adrenal glands is to produce adrenaline and that it is that hormone which prepares the body for 'fight or flight.' Many thousands of years ago this human response to stress and danger evolved during the struggle for survival in the African savannah.

We live in a rapidly changing and increasingly artificial world and although our lives are far removed from those of our distant ancestors we still have within us the inherited response to any sign of trouble. In our daily lives we are subject to any number of stresses and strains which may stimulate our adrenals to pump adrenaline into our system.

Even before we get to work we battle to get the kids out of bed and off to school on time, and when we fight through the crowds to get on the bus or the train, or suffer the aggressive behaviour of drivers on the road. It seems sometimes that every other person on the road is someone to be feared or challenged. As we all know, incidences of 'road rage' are on the increase and this phenomenon is a prime example of territorial behaviour inherited from our ancestors.

By nine o'clock in the morning there have been at least a dozen or so occasions when our adrenal systems have primed our bodies so it is no wonder that, as Dr Dalvi so aptly puts it, we are suffering from adrenal fatigue. They say that identifying the problem is half way to creating the solution so, by focussing on the problem, he has done not only the medical profession, but all of us who struggle through the daily round, an invaluable service. Not only that, but he has also come up with a number of practical and simple solutions, so he deserves our gratitude for that also.

Disclaimer:

The work that I have done and the information provided is with a view to educate and therefore every effort has been made to be as accurate and complete. I accept no liability nor responsibility to any person or entity with respect to any loss, damage or injury caused or alleged to be caused directly or indirectly by the information provided in my work. The information does not substitute medical consultation.

CONTENTS

INTRODUCTION

ADRENAL FATIGUE

One of the most common problems faced by men, women and children in modern times is stress. As a nutritional consultant I have been using the Bio Energetic stress system to monitor Hormonal irregularities, food intolerances and vitamin and mineral deficiencies. In eighteen months, I have seen over 500 clients in six countries and four continents and over 65% complain of being stressed, over tired or worn out and they just can't regain their energy, no matter how many doctors they visit or medications they take.

I was horrified at the number of stress cases and this led me to research what was the common underlying factor. I looked at my clients in UK, USA and South Africa and compared them with the clients from India, Kenya and Tanzania. I further subdivided them into two categories, rich and poor. My results were fascinating, all the stressed clients were from the industrialised well to do backgrounds. People from small towns, villages and those who led a non-aspiration life, were normally not stressed. Businessmen so called successful wealthy individuals and those who aspired for wealth were always stressed.

I investigated this group in detail and to my surprise all the stressed clients had adrenal hormone imbalance. I then visited many conventional doctors and practitioners, and asked them why Adrenal Fatigue was not commonly diagnosed or talked about. I was informed that the reason for this might be that there are not enough patentable treatments available.

I therefore decided, that I would take it upon myself to write about my findings and to increase awareness of Adrenal Fatigue and adrenal health.

CHAPTER ONE

The Adrenal Glands

The adrenal glands are located on top of the kidneys near the spine, just underneath the last rib. They are classified as endocrine glands as they secrete hormones directly into the bloodstream, influencing bodily processes including metabolism. The right adrenal gland is pyramid shaped and the left a semicircular half moon shape, they weigh between 3 to 5 grams. The adrenal glands of women are slightly lighter than those of men.

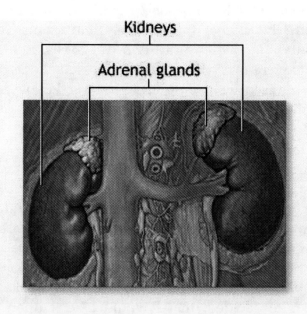

Function of the adrenal glands:

The adrenal glands work interactively with the hypothalamus and pituitary gland in the following process:

The hypothalamus produces corticotropin-releasing hormones, which stimulate the pituitary gland.

The pituitary gland, in turn, produces corticotropin hormones, which stimulate the adrenal glands to produce corticosteroid hormones.

Both parts of the adrenal glands -- the adrenal cortex and the adrenal medulla -- perform very separate functions.

What is the adrenal cortex?

The adrenal cortex, the outer portion of the adrenal gland, secretes hormones that have an effect on the body's metabolism, on chemicals in the blood, and on certain body characteristics. The adrenal cortex secretes corticosteroids and other hormones directly into the bloodstream. The hormones produced by the adrenal cortex include:

- **Corticosteroid hormones**

    o **Hydrocortisone hormone** - this hormone, also known as cortisol, controls the body's use of fats, proteins, and carbohydrates.

    o **Corticosterone** - this hormone, together with hydrocortisone hormones, suppresses inflammatory reactions in the body and also affects the immune system.

- **Aldosterone hormone** - this hormone inhibits the level of sodium excreted into the urine, maintaining blood volume and blood pressure.

- **Androgenic steroids (androgen hormones)** - these hormones have minimal effect on the development of male characteristics.

What is the adrenal medulla?

The adrenal medulla, the inner part of the adrenal gland, is not essential to life, but helps a person in coping with physical and emotional stress. The adrenal medulla secretes the following hormones:

- **Epinephrine (also called adrenaline)** - this hormone increases the heart rate and force of heart contractions, facilitates blood flow to the muscles and brain, causes relaxation of smooth muscles, helps with conversion of glycogen to glucose in the liver, and other activities.

- **Norepinephrine (also called noradrenaline)** - this hormone has little effect on smooth muscle, metabolic processes, and cardiac output, but has strong vasoconstrictive effects, thus increasing blood pressure.

-

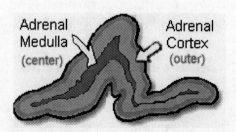

CHAPTER TWO

What is Adrenal Fatigue?

Adrenal Fatigue is a decreased ability of the adrenal glands to carry out their normal function. The main symptom of Adrenal Fatigue is tiredness accompanied by many other symptoms. Adrenal Fatigue occurs when stress from any source' whether emotional, physical, environmental or mental, exceeds either cumulatively in intensity the body's capacity to adjust properly to demands put on it by stress.

Is Adrenal Fatigue Common?

Yes, Adrenal Fatigue affects billions of people world wide, the problem is far more severe in industrialised, so called first world countries. My experience with clients in India, Tanzania and Kenya showed low signs of adrenal stress, however with my clients in United Kingdom and South Africa every second person showed Adrenal Fatigue to some extent.

Who Suffers from Adrenal Fatigue?

Anyone can suffer from Adrenal Fatigue, right from birth to old age regardless of sex, colour, race or culture. People vary in their ability to withstand stress and respond to it. However those people who suffer repeatedly from serious illness, infectious disease, allergies, malnutrition, intense emotional and physical pressure, or those who are exposed to toxic environment (such as nuclear medicine radiographers) are most likely to suffer from Adrenal Fatigue.

Children born to parents suffering Adrenal Fatigue may also suffer from the same condition. These children are often more sickly, and have less ability to handle stressful situations and take longer to recover from illness.

Once I have Adrenal Fatigue can I recover?

The answer to this question is simple and straight forward, with proper supervision and treatment most people can recover fully from Adrenal Fatigue.

What are the causes of Adrenal Fatigue?

There are multitude of causes of Adrenal Fatigue, but they usually stem from some common sources that overwhelm the body.

1. Diseases such as severe bronchitis or recurrent pneumonia, flu, diabetes, auto immune diseases, cancer and AIDS as well as other illnesses.
2. Physical stress such as surgery, poor nutritional habits, addiction, injury and exhaustion.
3. Emotional stress, usually arising from relationships, work or psychological origins.
4. Continual severe environmental stress from toxic chemicals, pollutants and prolonged use of medication.

Can age be a factor?

People of any age can suffer from Adrenal Fatigue however the very young and the very old are more vulnerable to stress and therefore can get Adrenal Fatigue.

How often can I suffer from Adrenal Fatigue?

This depends on the ability of a person to cope with a situation. In some instances people may only have one instance during a lifetime, however most of us have several experiences of chronic fatigue and we never fully recover.

Can Adrenal Fatigue be chronic?

In some people the adrenal glands do not fully recover because the stress was too great or prolonged or the person has general poor health.

However, even if there is chronic Adrenal Fatigue it will be because of factors that can normally be changed.

What is the difference between Hypoadrenia and Adrenal Fatigue?

Hypoadrenia is a medical term referring to adrenal failure or a completely low adrenal function. This condition is also called Addison disease. Less severe cases of Hypoadrenia are called Adrenal Fatigue.

Will I get more infections if I have Adrenal Fatigue?

Adrenal Fatigue sufferers in general have a decreased immune function and therefore are more at risk to illness and infections, such as infections of the respiratory tract.

Additionally people who are HIV positive or have Hepatitis C also have Adrenal Fatigue. The treatments for Hepatitis C is administration of corticosteroids drugs. These suppress the immune system and the adrenals. HIV sufferers have also shown compromised adrenal glands.

Can Allergies be associated with Adrenal Fatigue?

In my observation, people suffering with Adrenal Fatigue have a definitive increase in allergic response. This is because cortisol, the major adrenal hormone has a powerful anti-inflammatory action in the body. When a person has Adrenal Fatigue, their cortisol levels are low and hence the body has a more likely effect to have an increased allergic reaction (allergic reactions are inflammatory reactions) and these reactions will be more severe depending on the extent of the fatigue.

Does diet play a part in Adrenal Fatigue?

Diet has a lot to do with Adrenal Fatigue. Both the cause of the Adrenal Fatigue and the recovery from Adrenal Fatigue are diet related. Food intolerance and poor eating habits, such as fast foods, convenience meals, the time that we eat and how we chew our food are major causes for malabsorption of nutrients and lack of essential nutrients can put additional pressure on the adrenal glands.

In my experience whilst working with the BEST system Wheat, Milk and Egg intolerances are commonly prevalent.

It is therefore advisable to read the ingredient labels on products. However, as a guideline I have included two lists below to identify foods containing Wheat and Milk.

1. Products that contain wheat are: bran, wheat germ, wheat starch or gluten. Baked goods, Bagels, Biscuits, Bread crumbs, Bread, Breakfast cereals, Cakes, Coffee substitutes, Cookies, Cracker meal, Crackers, Doughnuts, Dumplings, Ice cream cones, sandwiches, Gravy, Hamburgers, Luncheon meats, Malt, Muffins, Pancakes, Pasta (macaroni, spaghetti, lasagna, etc.), Pies, Pizza, Salad dressing, Sauces that have been thickened but are opaque (e.g. cream sauce), Soups, Stuffing, Waffles

2. Products that contain milk are: Dried, condensed, evaporated or liquid whole, 2%, 1%, skim, lactase treated, acidophilus milk and buttermilk, Breaded meat, fish or

poultry, Butter, Casein or caseinate (milk protein), Cheese, Cream, Custard, Egg replacers, High calcium cereals, Ice cream, Omelettes, Scrambled eggs, Sour cream, Whey, Whipped topping, Yoghurt.

Constipation and irregular bowel movement can also affect Adrenal Fatigue.

Can exercise affect Adrenal Fatigue?

In my opinion too much exercise puts pressure on the adrenal glands and it is therefore better to exercise in moderation. If a person pushes their body through strenuous exercise, skips meals and eats so called meal replacements whilst training, this does not mean they are healthy. On the contrary they are testing the adrenal hormones and therefore significantly increasing their risk to Adrenal Fatigue.

Does smoking increase the risk of Adrenal Fatigue?

Any burden placed on the body requires the use of the adrenal glands. Smoking places additional stress on the lungs and respiratory tract and if the adrenals are already weak this can accelerate Adrenal Fatigue.

Does Adrenal Fatigue affect a person's sex life or a woman's menstrual cycle?

Pre menstrual syndrome, altered menstrual flow and menopause can definitely lead to Adrenal Fatigue. Decreased sex drive is also a common complaint related to Adrenal Fatigue. As the adrenals are responsible for manufacturing the sex hormones low adrenal function can lead to low performance and lack of desire in both men as well as women.

Does pregnancy lead to Adrenal Fatigue?

Generally speaking pregnancy helps Adrenal Fatigue recovery as the foetus produces a greater amount of natural adrenal hormone. However if the pregnancy is very stressful and the partners are not supportive of each other it can lead to Adrenal Fatigue.

Is there a connection between Hypoglycaemia and Adrenal Fatigue?

In order to answer this question we have first to look and understand the subject of Hypoglycaemia.

Hypoglycaemia (Low Blood Sugar)

What is hypoglycaemia?

Hypoglycaemia is the condition of having a glucose (blood sugar) level that is too low to effectively fuel the body's blood cells. Glucose is the main source of fuel for the body. The normal range of blood sugar is approximately 60 to 120 mg/dl (milligrams of glucose per decilitre of blood). When the level is below 45 mg/dl, a serious condition is suspected.

Hypoglycaemia may be a condition by itself, or may be a complication of diabetes or other disorders. It is most often seen as a complication of diabetes, which is sometimes referred to as insulin reaction.

What causes hypoglycaemia?

There are many different possible causes of hypoglycaemia, including:

- Diabetics taking too much insulin to lower the blood sugar

- Diabetics on insulin taking too little food in comparison to the units of insulin injected.

- Diabetics who miss a meal or exercise too strenuously

- Other drugs used to treat diseases such as AIDS-related pneumonia

- Psychological disturbances

- Alcohol consumption without eating adequately

- Insulin-producing tumour in the pancreas

What are symptoms of hypoglycaemia?

The following are the most common symptoms. However, each individual may experience symptoms differently. Symptoms may include:

- Shakiness

- Dizziness

- Sweating

- Hunger

- Headache

- Irritability

- Pale skin colour

- Sudden moodiness or behaviour changes, such as crying for no apparent reason

- Clumsy or jerky movements

- Difficulty paying attention, or confusion

- Tingling sensations around the mouth

Extremely low blood sugar can induce a coma. The symptoms of hypoglycaemia may resemble other conditions or medical problems. Consult a physician for diagnosis.

How is hypoglycaemia diagnosed?

In addition to a complete medical history and medical examination, diagnostic procedures for hypoglycaemia may include blood tests to measure blood sugar levels and insulin levels.

Treatment for hypoglycaemia:

Consuming sugar when experiencing symptoms of hypoglycaemia usually provides relief. Specific treatment for hypoglycaemia will be determined by your physician based on:

- Your overall health and medical history

- Extent of the disease

- Your tolerance for specific medications, procedures, or therapies

Treatment may also include taking glucagon, a protein hormone secreted by the pancreas to stimulate the liver to produce glucose. If the hypoglycaemia is a result of an insulin-producing tumour in the pancreas, the tumour is usually removed surgically. Chronic hypoglycaemia in persons without diabetes may benefit from eating frequent, small meals.

Can Hypoglycaemia cause Adrenal Fatigue?

There is a major link between hypoglycaemia (low blood sugar) and Adrenal Fatigue.

When the adrenals are fatigued, the cortisol output is reduced and the patient has lower levels of circulating blood cortisol. As cortisol is required for converting stored blood sugar in the liver to glucose (active blood sugar) lower cortisol will result in the diminished ability for the liver to complete conversion. Fats, Proteins and Carbohydrates other sources of glucose can also not be readily converted into active blood sugar. The adrenal hormones control these energy sources and hence healthy adrenal function is essential to achieving and maintaining normal blood sugar level especially during stress.

Additionally during stress the body increases insulin production, as there is an increased demand for energy. Without adequate cortisol levels to facilitate the conversion of glycogen, fats and protein to new glucose supplies, the increased demand is impossible to meet. This combination leads to low blood sugar production. To the body, hypoglycaemia is a strong stressor, an emergency call to further drain the already compromised adrenals. Low blood sugar also affects brain function.

The typical times for low blood sugar is mid morning and mid afternoon.

Is Adrenal Fatigue linked to chronic fatigue syndrome?

Adrenal Fatigue is a common, but usually not talked about as a component of chronic fatigue syndrome. The most likely connection is that factors that lead to the development of chronic fatigue also set up conditions that foster Adrenal Fatigue.

Is Adrenal Fatigue linked to clinical Depression and Fibromyalgia?

Mild depression is a sign of Adrenal Fatigue, in order to associate clinical depression to the adrenals we need to conduct certain clinical tests. Fibromyalgia sufferers however have compromised adrenal function.

Does Adrenal Fatigue affect the thyroid gland?

Although it is not widely reported, a sizeable majority of people suffering from adrenal exhaustion also suffer from decreased thyroid activity. The thyroid is another endocrine gland sensitive to the effects of stress. The main function of the thyroid gland is to control the rate at which energy is produced.

Often people who have an under active thyroid, have a sluggish metabolic rate. In order to correct the metabolic rate they are often prescribed medication to which they do not respond. In my opinion this is because they suffer from Adrenal Fatigue. For these people to get well, the adrenals must be supported in addition to the thyroid.

Is Sleep a factor?

Lack of sleep is a sign of either low or high cortisol levels and this can be a significant burden on the body and hence the adrenals. Continual lack of sleep leads to decreased immunity, impaired glucose tolerance, irritability and increases circulating estrogens levels, upsetting hormonal balance. Lack of sleep can also slow down the recovery process; it is therefore imperative one must sleep at least an average of six to eight hours a day.

Increased blood levels of stress hormones in people with chronic insomnia suggests these individuals suffer from sustained, round-the-clock activation of the body's system for responding to stress.

For this reason, the researchers suggest, doctors who treat insomnia should go beyond improving the quality or quantity of their patients' sleep and seek to **reduce this hyper arousal**, which is a risk factor for both psychiatric and medical illness.

Investigators monitored the sleep patterns of patients with insomnia and people without sleep disturbances (the "control" group). Blood was collected every 30 minutes for 24 hours, and levels of stress hormones -- adrenocorticotropic hormone (ACTH) and cortisol were monitored.

Average levels of both hormones were significantly higher in the insomniacs than in the control group.

They found that the insomniacs with the highest degree of sleep disturbance secreted the highest amount of cortisol, particularly in the evening and night time hours This means that insomniacs are experiencing hormonal changes in their bodies, which prevents them from sleeping.

CHAPTER THREE

What can I do to prevent Adrenal Fatigue?

Unlike other conditions, you can do what is necessary to recover and regain adrenal health yourself. There are no magic tablets that a doctor can prescribe for recovery of the adrenals. However, lifestyle changes and nutritional supplements can facilitate early recovery. Healing depends on how you spend your energy, how you conserve your energy and how you create energy. The second part is to do with nutrition, what you eat and drink and the thoughts you feed your mind and base your beliefs on. Therefore as a person who suffers from Adrenal Fatigue you have full control over your recovery.

RECOVERY FROM ADRENAL FATIGUE

Lifestyle is very important for Adrenal Fatigue recovery, removing the aggravating factors in most circumstances is the first step. The patient must decide what is good for them and what is bad for them. They must find out what are the energy robbers? Are they people you associate with or is it work or is it the home environment or is it food? Once these things have been identified, then begins the process of eliminating them and reducing the drain on the adrenals. There are three things one can do to stop energy drain a/ change the situation b/ you can adapt to the situation c/ you can leave the situation.

Let me quote an example, my wife keeps on telling me how unhappy she is at work and how difficult her employers, where the distance she was travelling every morning compounds and the traffic was affecting her. The choices to her to recovery from the fatigue are, either change her work, adapt to the situation or she can just ignore the situation. Although it would not be easy to ignore the situation and leave it, a decision has to be made, otherwise the body system would start to break down. The questions my wife had to deal with were:

1. Why was she working?
2. Was her career important to her?
3. What was wrong at work?
4. Was the travelling affecting her health?
5. Were all of the above affecting her marriage?

Once she had identified the reason for the drain it was very easy to decide which of the three alternatives she had and how she was going to reduce her stress levels.

There are other lifestyle areas that we need to look at briefly that help reduce stress level and help towards adrenal recovery.

Relaxation:

Learning to relax and take control of a situation is a way to adapt to difficult situations. Leisure activities are often thought of as a good relaxation exercise, however psychological relaxation is a set specific internal change that occurs when your body and mind are calm. It is definitely not the same as sleeping, rest or having fun, as although a person may be trying to entertain themselves by keeping away from a set of circumstances, their mind is not at rest and internal calm is not there, hence the body gets stressed even more.

To quote an example a person is having marital difficulties and they feel that in order to cope they will go out over the weekend or go on holiday. They may be having fun on the outside, but deep down they are always wondering about their partner and how it would have been if? This feeling is then exasperated by people around them giving opinions and views on the situation, so instead of relaxing they become stressed and confused. This makes it very difficult for adrenal recovery.

In order for the body to relax it has to change from a sympathetic to parasympathetic nervous system dominance, meaning the heart rate has to slow down, breathing must be relaxed, oxygen consumption is reduced comparatively and the brain generates slower wave patterns.

There are many effective ways to relax the body and some of these exercises include breathing from the belly, slowing down your breathing, prayer and meditation, progressive relaxation, and sleep.

FOOD

Diet and Adrenal Fatigue are closely related, as we already know from the question on hypoglycaemia or low blood sugar. It is very important therefore, for people with Adrenal Fatigue to eat, but it is equally important as to what they eat and the time they eat and how much water they consume.

People often eat fast foods and consume caffeine drinks to boost their energy; this temporarily increases cortisol levels and they feel fine but in the long run these people will have chronically low cortisol and thus put on weight. This is because excess cortisol causes fat to be deposited around the stomach area. Added weight leads to lethargy and the vicious cycle continues.

Another dietary mistake that people make is knowing when to eat, for example breakfast is the most important meal, because when you are asleep the bodies mechanisms use a lot energy and the glucose levels are low when one wakes up.

For those people who feel that they are not hungry in the

morning or cannot eat, it is advisable to seek help as their liver might be congested. Liver congestion does not mean that your body does not require the food and energy.

The second meal that I recommend is an early nourishing lunch, followed by a small snack at around 3pm as your cortisol and sugar levels sink mid afternoon. Evening meals should be eaten early and a small bite before bed is also advisable to avoid anxiety attacks during the night and get proper rest. It is also important to realise that if you feel dizzy during the day or like crashing out, it means Adrenal Fatigue and hypoglycaemia are creeping up on you and you have left it too late to eat.

In totality, if you suffer from Adrenal Fatigue, it is always recommended to combine fats, proteins and carbohydrates at every meal and snack. It is not advisable to have sugary food, or fruit juices as these raise blood sugar too quickly and subsequently fall too low, whereas starchy foods convert to sugar slowly and provide a steady source of energy.

There are many myths and diets that profess to help loose weight and to keep a person's body healthy. These diets and programmes may from time to time not cater for the total body picture stressing the adrenals. It is therefore very important when considering a healthy lifestyle to look at the types of food and why the body requires them.

Nutritional scientists and Biologists have classified foods into different components of energy, nutrients and fibres. The Energy portion is to get the body fuel, the nutrient is to get vitamins and minerals and fibre is to keep the bodily functions healthy.

In order to understand this further one must look at the basic types of food and how they are assimilated by the body to provide healthy functioning

Proteins

Quality Proteins such as meat, fish, eggs and dairy and legumes are essential to adrenal recovery. However, processed proteins must be avoided. Proteins when lightly cooked are easily digested and have more food, however it is advisable to fully cook meats because of microbial dangers. Once proteins are digested they form amino acids, which are responsible to form vital body structures and functions. Many people with Adrenal Fatigue need these amino acids however as their digestion is inadequate they cannot break down the proteins causing further stress and aggravating the condition.

The following Food Choice table indicates good and bad choice proteins.

	Good Choice	Reasons	Bad Choice	Reasons
Protein	Legumes	Soluble fibre	Peanuts	Aflatoxin (carcinogen)
	Nuts	High in Monounsaturated fats		
	Deep water fish	High in Omega 3 Fatty Acid	Coastal Fish	Toxic Metals
	Organic Eggs	Best Biological Value Protein for Human	Red Meats	Acid forming, Carcinogenic, Increase Hormone
	Nuts	Monounsaturated fatty acid (lower cholesterol), fibres	Dairy	Allergen, Hormone Increase
			Shellfish	Carcinogenic

LIPIDS

People with Adrenal Fatigue often crave fats and oils, partly because foods high in fats make them feel better for longer than low fat or sweet foods. Some fats also contain cholesterol needed by the adrenal glands to make the steroid hormones essential for adrenal activity throughout your body. Ideally lipids should not form more than quarter of your daily intake of foods. It is also very important that one consumes the right kind of fats, such as essential fatty acids which the body does not produce and is available from seeds and plants. Hydrogenated fats such as lard and butter must be kept to a minimum.

The following Food Choice table indicates good and bad choice fats

	Good Choice	Reasons	Bad Choice	Reasons
Fat	Avocado	Monounsaturated fatty acid (lower cholestrol)	Margarine	Hydrogenated Oil - carcinogenic
	Olive Oil	Monounsaturated fatty acid (lower cholestrol)	Deep Fried Food	Hydrogenated Oil - carcinogenic
	Polyunsaturated Oil when not heated	High in Omega 6 fatty acid	Chips	Hydrogenated Oil - carcinogenic
			Saturated Fats-Palm	Increase Cholestrol
			Polyunsaturated Oil when Heated	Hydrogenated Oil - carcinogenic
			Soft Drinks	Acidic, high sugar
			Desserts	High in sugar, high in hydrogenated fats
			Sugar	Empty calories, Increase TG, Inc Cholesterol, Dental Caries

CARBOHYDRATES

This group of foods is very broad and the body metabolises energy from them. Carbohydrates such as potatoes, cassava, yam, unrefined grains such as brown rice are normally regarded as a good source of carbohydrate, however, quick release carbohydrates such as sugar can be detrimental to adrenal as well as general health.

It is recommended to refer to the glycemic index of individual foods, before consuming them if you suffer from Adrenal Fatigue. The index only considers the extent to which the particular foods elevates blood sugar and is not concerned with the foods nutrient value as is a general misconception.

The following Food Choice table indicates good and bad choice carbohydrates.

	Good Choice	Reasons	Bad Choice	Reasons
Carbohydrates	Vegetables - green leafy	Vitamins, Minerals, Antioxidants, fibre	Most Tuber vegetables (potatoes, tapioca)	High glycemic index
	Onions, Green Onions, Chives, Garlic	Antibacterial, antiviral, anticarcinogenic		
	Cabbage, Broccoli, Cauliflower	Prevent estrogens dominance causing cancer.		
	Tomatoes (both raw and cook)	High Vitamin C and lycopene for CA prevention		
	Tubor vegetables in moderation - (carrots, beets, sweet potatoes)	Beta Carotene - good antioxidant		
	Whole Fruits -	Vitamins, Minerals, Antioxidants, fibre	Fruits (banana, Watermelon)	High glycemic index
	Lemon, Lime	Keep the body alkaline	Fruit Juices	High sugar content, low fibre
	Soybean Products in moderation	Cancer prevention		
	Pineapples	Bromelain		
	Blueberry, grapes	Protect the Heart		
	Whole Grains	B-Vitamins, Insoluble fibre		
	Oats, Barley	Soluble fibre, Lower Cholesterol	White Rice	High glycemic index
	Pasta made with durum wheat	Low to medium glycemic index	White Flour	High glycemic index
	Basmati Rice	Low glycemic index		

VEGETABLES

Raw vegetables provide vitamins, minerals, anti oxidants, Phyto- nutrients and fibre.

Its is advisable to have at least four to six portions of a wide variety of vegetables in your daily intake of food. In some cases it may be advisable to cook vegetables, where the heat releases the vitamin or anti oxidant (Carrots--- release caratonoid Vit A, Tomatoes--- for Lycopene). Seed and Bean sprouts are also very rich in quality nutrients and help Adrenal recovery.

THE ACT OF EATING AND ADRENAL RECOVERY

How you eat can have as much effect on adrenal recovery as what you eat.

Before you begin a meal, it is important to prepare your body so that it too can begin the complicated process of digestion, absorption and utilisation of energy and nutrients. It is always advisable to choose pleasant peaceful surroundings and think of enjoyable things that relax you, so as to promote relaxation and digestion.

Rushing through a meal while focusing on work problems, and eating with people who make you tense, leads to the food not being digested properly, leading either to fermentation or putrefaction of the food. It is also good to eat your food whilst sitting down in one place and once you have sat down to take a few deep breaths so as to relax and calm the body before beginning to eat.

Chewing the food well makes a significant difference on how well the food is digested. This allows the enzymes that are in the mouth to properly mix with the food and begin the breakdown of the food and also promotes relaxation.

In my opinion it is also advisable to avoid consuming water or beverages half an hour either side of a meal. Consumption of beverages may dilute the digestive juices and that may contribute to stress. Additionally, caffeine rich beverages over stimulate the adrenals temporarily and eventually lead to excessive Adrenal Fatigue.

THE ROLE OF WATER IN ADRENAL RECOVERY AND THE BODY

Water performs many essential functions in the human body. One of the primary functions is to provide shape by exerting fluid pressure on the cell membranes. The Female body is approximately 50 to 55 percent water, while the male body is 55 to 65 percent water. The higher water content in most men is due to their muscle content. Water makes up about three fourths of the weight of lean tissue and less than one fourth of the weight of fat. Therefore if a person weighs 165 pounds, he will be carrying approximately 90 to 105 pounds of water.

Water serves as a medium for all life, supporting chemical reactions in the body. The reason for this is that it is the necessary chemical solvent on which various body tissue solutions are based. Water also maintains stable body temperature.

Depending on the climate, the skin will adjust its water loss in order to maintain an acceptable body temperature.

As perspiration is evaporated, the body is cooled. Water is also important in maintaining blood volume, carrying nutrients and waste products throughout the body, and acting as a lubricant and cushion around joints and other areas of the body, such as inside the eyes.

Risk Factors and Symptoms

The primary safeguard against dehydration is the thirst mechanism. Thirst occurs as a result of even small fluid losses. As we age, the thirst mechanism becomes less sensitive, and many elderly and infirm patients may not even recognize thirst, due to altered cognition or sensory impairments. Other risk factors for dehydration include Adrenal Fatigue, stress, diarrhoea, fever, uncontrolled diabetes, dementia, fluid restrictions, diuretic therapy, and functional impairments, such as not being able to hold a drinking cup, urinary tract infections, internal bleeding, and swallowing disorders. When a patient is assessed as having one or more risk factors for dehydration, it is important to be able to recognize the symptoms of dehydration and have an action plan.

Symptoms of Dehydration

Symptoms of moderate-to-severe dehydration include:

- Low blood pressure
- Fainting
- Severe muscle contractions in the arms, legs, stomach, and back
- Convulsions
- A bloated stomach
- Heart failure
- Lack of urine output
- Sunken, dry eyes with few or no tears
- Skin without firmness that looks wrinkled
- Lack of elasticity and tenting of the skin (when a bit of skin is lifted up, it stays folded and takes a long time to return to its normal position)
- Rapid and deep breathing
- Fast, weak pulse

Symptoms of early or mild dehydration include:

- Flushed Face
- Extreme thirst or inability to drink
- Dry, warm skin
- Cannot pass urine or passing reduced amounts of dark yellow urine
- Dizziness made worse when standing
- Weakness
- Cramping in the arms and legs
- Crying with few or no tears
- Sleepy or irritable
- Unwell
- Headaches
- Dry mouth and/or dry tongue with thick saliva

Estimating Fluid Needs

It is often said that we need to drink twelve glasses of water each day. While this is a good general rule, more precise estimates of fluid needs may be based on caloric intake or body weight. This is because the requirement is the amount necessary to balance the insensible losses (which can vary markedly) and maintain a tolerable solute load for the kidneys (which may vary with dietary composition and other factors). Rather than set a Recommended dietary allowance (RDA)

For water, the NAS/NRC advises that 1ml/kcal of energy expenditure can be recommended as the water requirement for adults. As with most recommendations, this is for adults under average conditions of activity and in average climates. The recommendation may be increased to 1.5ml/kcal to cover variations in activity level, sweating, and solute load.

The second method of estimation is based on body weight. For patients with normal fluid status, 30ml/kg of body weight is recommended. The estimate may range from 25-35 ml/kg body weights depending on the clinical condition of the individual. For example, a patient with congestive heart failure would require 25-ml/kg body weights, while a dehydrated patient would be assessed at the higher end of the range. It is important to note that the minimum recommendation regardless of caloric intake or weight is 1500ml/day.

Re-hydration Plan

The prevention and treatment of dehydration is the responsibility of the entire care team. Dehydration can begin in only a few hours, so it is important to constantly monitor for the warning signs. Carers should be trained to have a heightened awareness of dehydration, particularly in the warmer months. This can be accomplished within service education programs, listing the signs and symptoms for which to watch. Most treatment plans focus on providing a wide array of beverage choices at frequent intervals throughout the day. Although water is always a good choice, fluids may also include juice, milk, ice chips, fruit ices, soups, ice cream, and medical nutrition supplements, such as shakes. Foods with high water content may also contribute to the overall daily fluid intake. Caffeinated and alcoholic beverages must not be consumed, because they may have a diuretic effect.

CHAPTER FOUR

SUPPLEMENTS AND ADRENAL RECOVERY

It is my view that supplements play a major part in the role of healing from Adrenal Fatigue. They not only speed up the recovery process, but also are often essential to the recovery programme. I have studied and worked with a number of supplements which are specific for the restoration of the adrenal glands and are essential as part of a rehabilitation programme. The formulation that I personally formulated for **Bioharmony** and named **Adrenal Boost** is a combination of some of these supplements in therapeutic doses.

VITAMIN C

Vitamin C is probably the most important of all the vitamins, minerals and herbs required in adrenal recovery. The more we use the adrenal hormone cortisol the more the need for Vitamin C. It is also important for the manufacture of adrenal steroid hormone Vitamin C is also used all along the adrenal cascade and acts as a powerful antioxidant within the adrenal cortex.

Vitamin C is a composite of ascorbic acid and bioflavanoids and it is this combination that has the beneficial effects. Ascorbic acid cannot be fully metabolised without Bioflavanoids in the ration of two parts of the former to one part of the latter. Most supplements of Vitamin C available on the market worldwide are synthesised from corn syrup and others from cane or beet sugar. This does not mean that corn syrup, sugar or beet contain Vitamin C, it only means that they are the raw materials in the commercial production of Vitamin C. It is my view that people who have food sensitivities to corn, should check the source of the supplement.

As Vitamin C is water soluble and quickly used up by the body or excreted, it can be consumed in fairly regular doses several times a day. I cannot say that there is a specific dose for Vitamin C as the requirement varies from person to person. The dose will also vary if one is under stress either physical or emotional, or the body is fighting infections.

As a tip to those people who want to know how much Vitamin C is required by their individual body, there is a simple test. It is often called the loading test whereby you start with an initial dose of 500mg of Vitamin C complex, and keep increasing the dose by 500mg every hour until you get a runny bowel movement. Once you have got a runny bowel movement you reduce the dose by 500mg. This is then your optimum dose. Most of the people who I have suggested the above method of determining a therapeutic dose for Adrenal Fatigue, have a common point of between 2000mg to 4000mg daily. However many ND's have worked with between 15-20 grams daily in severe and chronic illnesses. One must also note that if you begin taking high doses of Vitamin C, the body adapts to higher levels and hence when one wants to reduce the dose it must be done gradually. Patients who are on anticoagulant or blood clotting medication, must exercise caution and Vitamin C should only be taken under medical supervision.

Vitamin C is commonly associated with the stimulation of the immune system. Everyone starts taking Vitamin C as soon as winter comes round, or as soon as there is the slight sign of a cold or infection. This is because as soon as there is a change in the body's normal circumstances a stressful situation develops and the adrenals are required to perform, so Vitamin C not only aids your immune system in fighting the infection it also helps the adrenals in responding to the stressful situation. I normally suggest that everyone takes Vitamin C regardless of whether they are under emotional stress or pushing themselves at work or school.

In my opinion and discussions with fellow professionals, if you do not avail your body of enough Vitamin C, the adrenal glands cannot make additional adrenal hormone required to maintain during stressful times. This means Adrenal Fatigue recovery is slower.

Fruits and green leafy vegetables and sprouted seeds such as Alfalfa are a rich food source of Vitamin C, however the amount available in the portions consumed is not sufficient for therapeutic dosages. I do however, recommend eating tomatoes, peppers, bananas, grapes and freshly picked oranges.

At this juncture I feel I must make clear that there is a myth regarding Vitamin C in oranges and orange juice. In the opinion of experts, unless you are living on a farm and eat freshly picked oranges the amount of Vitamin C available will be little or negligible. The reason for this, is that once Oranges are picked the Vitamin C and the bioflavanoids present in the orange will be used by the fruit itself for self protection and survival and because Vitamin C dissipates with time, by the time it gets to our shelves its too late. Same is the case with Orange juice, from harvest to manufacture to the table, the time is far too long for there to be any real Vitamin C.

Additionally it is not advisable for people suffering from Adrenal Fatigue to consume orange juice, especially at breakfast as this is again a quick solution to raise blood glucose levels which fall rapidly once the day has begun, making you feel more tired.

AMLA

Amla or Indian gooseberry, is known for its richest source of Vitamin C and gallic acid and bioflavanoids. The fruit is native to India and has been used by Ayurvedic and Unani physicians alike, for its immune enhancing and anti ageing properties. The fruit is said to help in protein assimilation as well as having a tonic effect on the adrenal glands and helps deal with stress. According to Unani physicians, a tablespoon of fresh Amla juice gives as much Vitamin C as nine kilos of medium size oranges, or eighteen kilos of grapes. Amla extract is therefore a valuable tool in adrenal recovery.

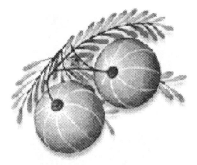

Amlica Embellicus

Vitamin E

Technically Vitamin E is not required for the manufacture of adrenal hormones, yet it is essential, as it indirectly required for its free radical scavenging properties. The manufacture of Adrenal hormones releases a lot of free radicals and these can damage cells. Vitamin E absorbs and neutralises these free radical molecules. Vitamin C and E also work hand in hand to keep the adrenals functioning at optimal levels. Vitamin E is also a natural blood thinning agent and anti – coagulant; patients must therefore consult a medical professional to determine their optimal dose and monitor blood clotting.

I have always suggested taking 800IU of mixed tocopherol brand of Vitamin E as beta tocopherols are also as essential in adrenal rejuvenation. In order to see significant results and adrenal recovery Vitamin E must be taken for at least 12 weeks. Vitamin E has other beneficial effects in the body and therefore continual use is also necessary so as to delay ageing.

VITAMIN B5

Vitamin B5 or Panthotenic acid is an essential contributor to the adrenal cascade. The combination of B5 with magnesium, Vitamin E and C increases energy production and relives the fatigue from the adrenal glands, without over stimulating them. The typical dosage is about 1500mg daily for about three months.

NIACIN

Niacin Vitamin B3 is also important in the manufacturing of adrenal hormones. Large amounts of this vitamin are required to facilitate some of the crucial enzymatic reactions. It is normally recommended that 20mg of non flushing niacin is taken for adrenal recovery.

Vitamin B6

In recent years we have seen many controversies regarding this important vitamin. Vitamin B6 is typically associated with premenstrual syndrome however, it is also a co -factor in several of the enzymatic pathways in the adrenal cascade. In premenstrual syndrome, stress is a high factor hence the adrenals are compromised. The typical therapeutic dose would be 50 to 100mg of B6 daily.

Vitamin B12 (Cobalamin):

Helps in the formation and regeneration of red blood cells and nerve tissue, helps in utilization of fats, proteins and carbohydrates. Promotes growth of children and a general tonic for adults. Deficiency may lead to anaemia and fatigue. The natural sources are milk products, meats, eggs, and liver.

The typical daily requirement 6.0 micrograms.

B Complex

In my opinion a complex of Vitamin B is not as essential for adrenal recovery as the quantities in any complex would not be in the correct proportions.

CALCIUM

The mineral calcium is associated with bones and bone building, however, one of the other functions of this mineral is to help calm the nervous system. Contrary to many of the theories it is best to take calcium separately from magnesium and as both minerals are best absorbed at night, it is recommended in my view to take them on alternate nights. The typical recommended amount is 750mg   calcium citrate on alternate nights. Although calcium carbonate is relatively cheap it is not absorbed easily.

Organic cows milk is a source of calcium, however the milk that we get commercially has been pasteurised denaturing the calcium and making it more difficult to absorb, additionally adding synthetic Vitamin D2 to milk produced a tendency for the calcium to be deposited on joints, instead of being made available in other parts of the body.
I normally suggest fish such as whitebait, sesame seeds, deep green vegetables, nuts and beans as an additional food source.

A calm and settled nervous system is stress free and the adrenals are therefore able to recover fairly rapidly.

Magnesium

Magnesium is the catalyst for both adrenal function and for the energy portion in every cell of the body. Magnesium works in conjunction with Vitamin C and Vitamin B5 to potentate the actions of the adrenals. Approximately 400mg of magnesium citrate is recommended daily. Although I have previously suggested that Calcium and magnesium should be taken on alternate nights, magnesium can be taken daily for adrenal recovery, or during times of high stress. Nutrition lists suggest magnesium is taken with acidic drinks such as tomato juice for optimal absorption.

Phosphorus

Phosphorous is needed for normal bone and tooth structure, inter-related with action of calcium and Vitamin D. It is also needed by certain key enzymes, which help change food into energy. It is also involved in many varied chemical reactions in the body. Its deficiency results in general weakness, bone pain and decreased appetite. Whole grain bread, beans, pulses, fish, poultry and meat are significant sources of this mineral.

Trace Minerals

Trace minerals such as chromium, zinc manganese, selenium and iodine also play a part in adrenal recovery, by having a calming effect on the body. This is especially valuable when Adrenal Fatigue is as a result of a trauma or accident. Trace minerals must also be taken before bed with an acidic juice.

I have so far identified vitamins that aid adrenal recovery, however in conjunction with these vitamins certain herbs also play a major and beneficial role.

HERBS

ASTRALAGUS

Astragalus's is a adaptogenic herb native to China, it contains a number of components that studies, and Chinese medical practitioners believe may restore immune activity. It has also been said that adaptogen such as Astragalus's are helpful in protecting the body against negative effects of long term stress. In terms of Chinese medication the herb is used to combat deficiency of chi e.g as in fatigue, loss of appetite or weakness, all common in Adrenal Fatigue.

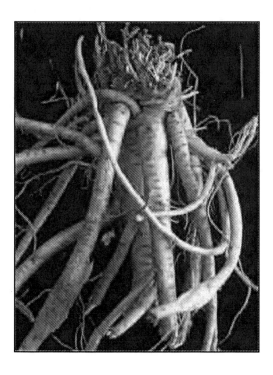

ASHWAGHANDA

Ashwaghanda or withania somnifera, is an ancient India herb with therapeutic benefits to the adrenal glands. The herb has been used by Ayurvedic practitioners in normalising cortisol levels, thus it is exceptionally beneficial in treating Adrenal Fatigue and supporting general recovery. Caution must however, be exercised as to the amount of Ashwaghanda used in treatment, as excessively high dosage of 35 grams or over can inhibit adrenal function.

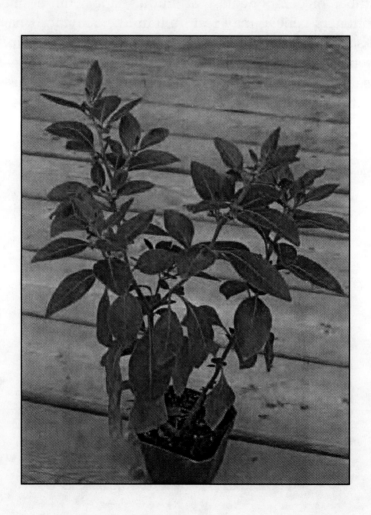

GINGER

Ginger root is another adaptogen that helps adrenal modulate cortisol levels. Ginger is also helpful in normalising blood pressure and heart rate, it is an excellent fat burner, helping lower cholesterol levels and increases metabolic function, thus energy levels. Ginger is also stimulates digestive enzyme secretion for the breakdown of protein and fatty acids. The herb is used in convalescence as well for morning sickness during pregnancy. Recently studies have demonstrated that *African Ginger* is also an immuno stimulant, antibiotic, as well as an anti-inflammatory.

This makes ginger very useful herb in the overall body maintenance.

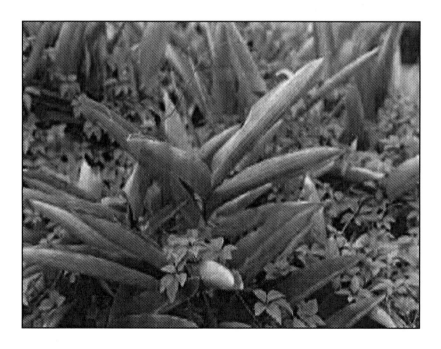

PIPER NIGRUM

Black Pepper has been used in Asian medication to fight free radical scavenging and studies demonstrate it prevents Glutathione depletion. Glutathione is an antioxidant involved in many cellular functions such as detoxification, amino acid transport, production of coenzymes and recycling of Vitamin E and C. It is therefore regarded as an essential detoxifier and helps certain enzymatic functions in the adrenal cascade.

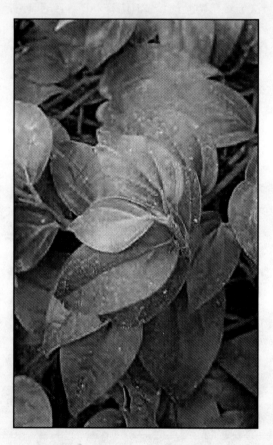

GINKGO LEAF

Ginkgo leaf is a powerful antioxidant in its own right and sequesters free radical production. When the adrenals are under stress they suffer tremendous oxidation especially when producing excessive cortisol, this produces free radicals. Ginkgo therefore acts as a protector for the adrenals in addition to its normal association to protect the brain and liver by increasing blood flow. It is important to know that Ginkgo also contains bioflavanoids that are responsible for the improved oxygenated blood flow.

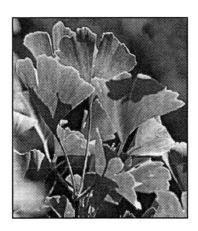

ROOIBOS

Rooibos or Red Bush is a herb native to the Western Cape region of South Africa. It has grown in popularity over the past decade due to its health properties. However, one of its indigenous uses was to treat nervousness. Recent studies however, have identified other potent antioxidant properties of this herb; these studies also identified a unique flavanoid Asphalatin which regarded to be more potent as an antioxidant than both Vitamin C and E. The primary function of Asphalatin is to prevent the body from attacking itself and additionally defending against external factors. As Rooibos also contains the minerals selenium and magnesium, in addition to the Vitamin A, C, E it is very useful in adrenal recovery. There have been many claims that the benefits of Rooibos as a tea, out weigh the benefits of it in an extract form. However from what I understand, the unique process used by Afriplex in South Africa make the capsule extract six times more powerful than a cup of tea.

Rooibos has other secondary benefits including age related brain deterioration, anticarcinogenis and anti HIV activity.

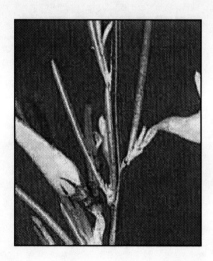

SUTHERLANDIA

Sutherlandia as a herb is growing in its popularity as a traditional herbal remedy. Although the herb has been used for over 100 year in South Africa, its popularity as a herb is due to the work done by the likes of **Dr. Nigel Gericke MD,** and the initial work done by **Foremost Supplements in the UK.**

Sutherlandia powerfully assists the body to mobilise its own immunological and physiological resources to combat disease, as well as physical and mental stress. It has demonstrated immunomudalatory, anti-inflammatory, and vasodilator. Analgesic, anti viral, anti fungal, anti- cancer properties and is also used in the treatment of AIDS patients. Amongst other components Sutherlandia also has the neurotransmitter **GABA** known for its beneficial effects on relaxation, stress and promoting sleep.

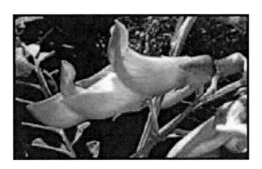

There are other herbs such as Ginseng both Siberian and Korean and Liquorice that have beneficial effects on adrenal recovery. However I am of the opinion that the contra indications associated with them far outweigh the benefits. In saying that I do not say that one must not take them but merely caution must be exercised.

HERBS THAT MAY HARM

Just as we have seen herbs can help adrenal recovery, there are certain herbs that can do exactly the opposite. These herbs include Ephedra or MaHuang, and Cola these over stimulate nervous system temporarily and give a false sense of euphoria.

FIBRE AND PRO BIOTICS

We have previously, already determined that people with Adrenal Fatigue have a compromised digestive system. This can mean that they are mildly constipated, and may have symptoms of yeast over growth.

Increasing the amount of fibre in your diet not only improves bowel movement, it also improves and strengthens adrenal function.

As the adrenals begin to recover the body systems become more efficient and the liver begins a process of detoxification or deamination. This process results in toxins being eliminated by the liver into the intestinal tract for elimination. Fibre binds with these toxins and moves them along the digestive tract for rapid elimination. Without sufficient fibres the toxins would be reabsorbed through the intestines.

There are two types of fibres; one, water soluble found in nuts, legumes, apples, oats and barley etc. which lowers cholesterol and blood fats and controls blood sugar levels and second, water insoluble fibre found in bran, whole grains and vegetables which controls constipation.

There are many fibres on the market, however I normally recommend Psyllium husks as a good bulking agent.

Probiotics are favourable lactic acid producing bacteria in the intestine that inhibit the growth of harmful bacteria, promote good digestion and boost immune function and increase resistance to infection. The most common Probiotics are Acidophilus and bifidobacteria; they produce compounds such as lactic acid, hydrogen peroxide and substances called bacteriocins, which act as natural antibiotics to kill undesirable microorganisms. Regular ingestion of probiotic may prevent virginal and intestinal yeast infection. Probiotics are therefore also a vital aid in an adrenal recovery programme.

Glutamine

Glutamine is normally the most abundant amino acid in the human body. However its importance in adrenal recovery is important, because it acts as a precursor of Glutathione, which is involved in many cellular functions as an antioxidant. Additionally, when the body is pushed e.g athletes the adrenals are fatigued as the muscles tire after a hard work out as a result of lactic acid build up in muscle cells. Supplementing with Glutamine reduces lactic acid build up and hence the muscles and adrenals are not stressed.

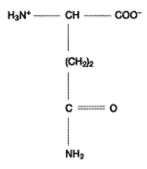

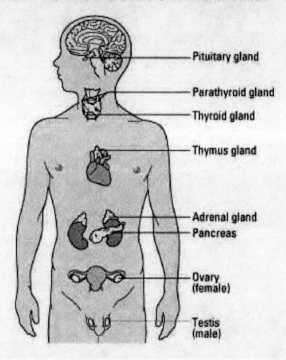

The Endocrine System
Glands which release chemicals directly into the blood stream.

Pituitary gland

Parathyroid gland

Thyroid gland

Thymus gland

Adrenal gland

Pancreas

Ovary
(female)

Testis
(male)

Glossary

ACTH: Adrenocorticotropic Hormone. ACTH is a normal by-product of the anterior pituitary gland. It acts by controlling the secretion of the adrenal hormone, cortisol. Produced by the pituitary gland.

Addison's Disease (Adrenal insufficiency): Caused by low levels of cortisone like hormones produced by the adrenal glands.

Adrenal glands – two glands that sit above the kidneys, responsible for the body's adaptation to stress.

Adrenal cortex - the outer portion of the adrenal gland that secretes hormones that are vital to the body.

Androgen hormone - a hormone secreted by the adrenal cortex, which affects blood pressure and saline balance.

Aldosterone - a hormone secreted by the adrenal cortex, which affects blood pressure and saline balance.

Blood Pressure: Constant force placed on the walls of the arteries.

Basal metabolic rate (BMR) - a measurement of energy required to keep the body functioning at rest. Measured in calories, metabolic rates increase with exertion, stress, fear, and illness.

Calcitonin - a hormone secreted by the thyroid gland which controls the levels of calcium and phosphorous in the blood.

Computed tomography (CT or CAT scan) - a non-invasive procedure that takes cross-sectional images of the brain or other internal organs; to detect any abnormalities that may not show up on an ordinary x-ray.

Corticosteroids - hormones produced by the adrenal gland, consisting of hydrocortisone and corticosterone.

Cholesterol: A waxy, fat-like substance contained in every cell in the body and in many foods. Some cholesterol in the blood is necessary - but a high level can lead to heart disease.

Chronic: Term used to describe long-lasting diseases or conditions. Usually, a chronic disease will last in some form for the remainder of the patient's life.

Estrogens - a hormone secreted by the ovaries, which affect many aspects of the female body, including menstrual cycles and pregnancy.

Glucagon - a protein hormone secreted by the pancreas to stimulate the liver to produce glucose.

Gonads - ovaries and testes.

Gonadotropins - luteinizing hormone and follicle-stimulating hormone, produced by the pituitary gland.

Gland: Any organ or tissue that releases a substance to be used elsewhere in the body; endocrine glands release hormones directly into the bloodstream.

Gonadotropins: A collective term for follicle stimulating hormone (FSH) and luteinizing hormone (LH).

Hormones - chemical substances created by the body that control numerous body functions.

Hydrocortisone - a hormone secreted by the adrenal cortex, which affects metabolism.

Hypothalamus - the portion of the brain that stimulates the pituitary gland.

Hypoglycaemia: Hypoglycaemia, or low blood sugar, occurs when blood levels of glucose drop too low to fuel the body's activity.

Insulin - a hormone released by the pancreas in response to increased levels of sugar in the blood.

Islets of Langerhans - pancreas cells that produce insulin and glucagon -- important regulators of sugar metabolism.

Magnetic resonance imaging (MRI) - a non-invasive procedure that produces two-dimensional view of an internal organ or structure, especially the brain and spinal cord.

Metabolism - the chemical activity that occurs in cells, releasing energy from nutrients or using energy to create other substances, such as proteins.

Oxytocin - a hormone secreted by the pituitary gland, which plays a role in childbirth.

Progesterone - a hormone secreted by the ovaries, which affect many aspects of the female body, including menstrual cycles and pregnancy.

Prolactin - a hormone secreted by the pituitary gland that affects growth of the mammatory glands.

Radioisotope scan - uses radioactive substances introduced into the body to create an image of the functioning adrenal gland.

Thyroid scan - uses a radioactive substance to create an image of the thyroid as it is functioning.

Thyroxin (T4) - a hormone secreted by the thyroid gland that regulates metabolism.

Triiodothyronine (T3) - a hormone secreted by the thyroid gland that regulates metabolism.

Ultrasound - a diagnostic technique that uses high-frequency sound waves to create an image of the internal organs.

X-ray - electromagnetic energy used to produce images of bones and internal organs onto film.

REFERENCES

1. Roberts SE. Exhaustion; Causes And Treatments. Emmaus, Penna 18049:Rodale Books, Inc
2. Journal of Ethno Pharmacology 1994
3. The American Journal of Physiology.
4. Physicians Desk reference
5. Dr. Whitakers Guide to natural healing. Prima Publishing Inc.
6. Prescriptions for nutritional Healing Avery Publishing 1990
7. Sports Nutrition Update 'Lets Live ' Sept 1997
8. Biology a functional Approach M.B.V Roberts M.A. P.H.D. third edition 1982
9. Adrenal Fatigue ... James Wilson ND. Smart Publications April 2001
10. Medicinal secrets of your food ...Dr. Aman 1988
11. Joubert E, Ferreira D. Antioxidants of Rooibos tea... SA journal of Food Science and Nutrition 1996
12. Antioxidant activity of Rooibos Tea ... Von Gadow A 1996
13. Peoples Plants – A guide to useful plants in South Africa Van Wyk and B.E Nigel Gericke Briza... Pretoria 2000
14. Journal of parental and Enteral Nutrition Hurson M et al Journal 1995
15. Positive Health Magazine issue number 85 Feb 2003
16. Planetary Herbology... Michael Tierra, C.A. N.D. LOTUS PRESS 1988
17. Journal of Clinical Endocrinology & Metabolism August 2001; 86:3787-3794
18. About Your Glands and Alcoholism John W. Tintera , 1958
19. The complete handbook of nutrition, Gary Null Steve Null, Robert Speller & Sons, 1972
20. Nutrition in Practice, volume 4, issue2. July 2003

INDEX

Printed in the United States
100344LV00003B/421-423/A

9 780755 200931